Evaluation of Environmental Controls at a Homeless Shelter (Trinity Rescue Mission) Associated with a Tuberculosis Outbreak – Florida

Stephen B. Martin, Jr., MS, PE
Kenneth R. Mead, PhD, PE
R. Brent Lawrence, MS, GSP
Michael C. Beaty

I0426205

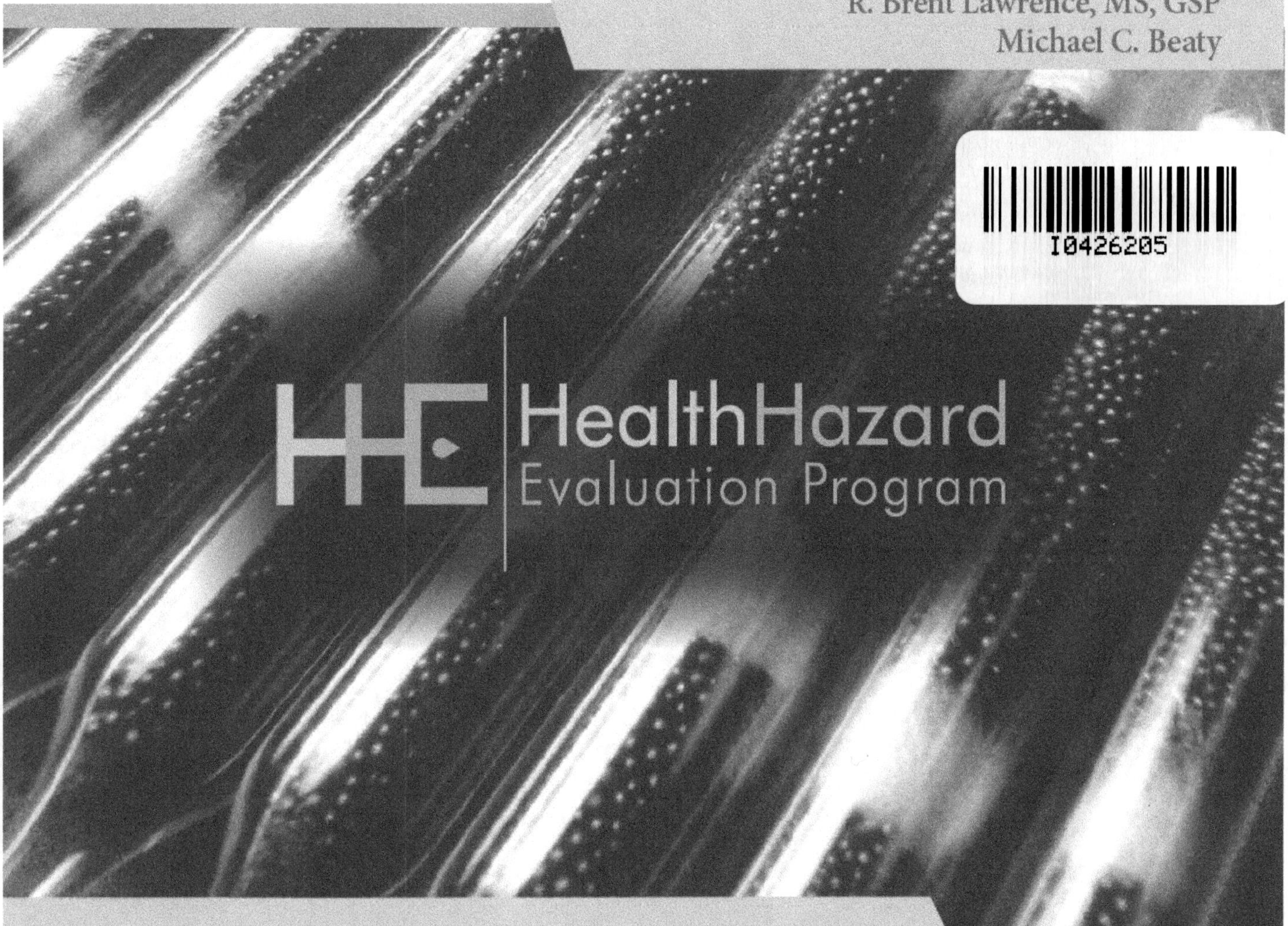

HealthHazard
Evaluation Program

Report No. 2012-0265-3183
July 2013

U.S. Department of Health and Human Services
Centers for Disease Control and Prevention
National Institute for Occupational Safety and Health

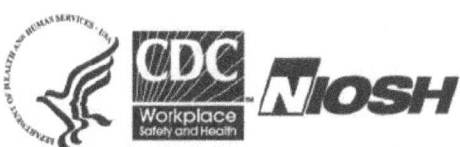

Contents

Highlights of this Evaluation

The National Institute for Occupational Safety and Health received a technical assistance request from the Duval County Health Department in Florida. The request asked that we assess the heating, ventilation, and air-conditioning systems and make recommendations to improve overall environmental controls at Trinity Rescue Mission, a local homeless shelter with epidemiological links to an ongoing tuberculosis outbreak.

What NIOSH Did

- We visited Trinity Rescue Mission on August 23, 2012.

- We met with representatives from the Duval County Health Department to discuss the ongoing tuberculosis outbreak.

- We recorded the physical sizes of occupied spaces.

- We measured ventilation air flow into/from occupied spaces.

- We collected information on all shelter air-handling units.

What NIOSH Found

- Trinity Rescue Mission did not have administrative controls in place to identify guests on priority screening lists or those with symptoms of tuberculosis.

- The shelter was not working closely with the Duval County Health Department on outbreak response efforts.

- Air-handling units were generally in good working order, but some had improper filter configurations and low-efficiency filters.

- No fresh outdoor air was being supplied to the occupied spaces by building mechanical systems.

- There were no clearly defined areas to separate guests suspected of having tuberculosis from the general guest population.

- Clinic examination rooms in the women's facility were incorrectly operating under positive pressure compared to the adjacent waiting area.

- A written respiratory protection plan did not exist.

- Some bathroom exhaust fans were not functional.

What Trinity Rescue Mission Should Do

- Work in close conjunction with the Duval County Health Department to improve overall administrative controls and help ensure rapid identification of guests suspected to have tuberculosis.

- Develop and implement a comprehensive infection control plan with input from the Duval County Health Department and Florida Department of Health.

- Modify or augment shelter ventilation systems to provide adequate fresh outdoor air to all occupied spaces using a strategy compatible with existing system capacities.

- Strategically reposition supply and exhaust grill locations to improve air flow patterns in occupied spaces, particularly in the three large guest sleeping areas.

- Install the highest efficiency air filters possible that is consistent with the proper operation of each air-handling unit.

- Modify at least one area in each of the men's and women's shelters for alternate use as respiratory separation areas.

- Install a properly designed upper-room ultraviolet germicidal irradiation system in the men's barracks-style sleeping area.

- Make ventilation changes to properly maintain medical examination rooms under negative pressure relative to the waiting area.

- Develop and implement a written respiratory protection program that meets the requirements of the Occupational Safety and Health Administration's respiratory protection standard 29 Code of Federal Regulations 1910.134.

- Repair or replace all bathroom exhaust fans which are not functioning properly.

- Develop and implement a written operation and maintenance plan for shelter heating, ventilation, and air-conditioning systems, to include a filter replacement schedule.

Abbreviations

μm	Micrometer
AHU(s)	Air-handling unit(s)
ACGIH	American Conference of Governmental Industrial Hygienists
ACH	Air changes per hour
AII	Airborne infection isolation
ANSI®	American National Standards Institute
ASHRAE®	American Society of Heating, Refrigerating and Air-Conditioning Engineers
CDC	Centers for Disease Control and Prevention
cfm	Cubic feet per minute
CFR	Code of Federal Regulations
DCHD	Duval County Health Department
DRDS	Division of Respiratory Disease Studies
DTBE	Division of Tuberculosis Elimination
FGI	Facility Guidelines Institute
HEPA	High-efficiency particulate air
HVAC	Heating, ventilation, and air-conditioning
ICP	Infection control plan
μW/cm2	Microwatts per square centimeter
mJ/cm2	Millijoules per square centimeter
MERV	Minimum efficiency reporting value
nm	Nanometer
NCHHSTP	National Center for HIV/AIDS, Viral Hepatitis, STD, and TB Prevention
NIOSH	National Institute for Occupational Safety and Health
O&M	Operation and maintenance
OSHA	Occupational Safety and Health Administration
REL	Recommended Exposure Limit
RH	Relative humidity
TB	Tuberculosis
UV	Ultraviolet
UVGI	Ultraviolet germicidal irradiation

Mention of any company or product does not constitute endorsement by NIOSH. In addition, citations to websites external to NIOSH do not constitute NIOSH endorsement of the sponsoring organizations or their programs or products. Furthermore, NIOSH is not responsible for the content of these websites. All web addresses referenced in this document

Summary

In May 2012, the National Institute for Occupational Safety and Health (NIOSH) received a request for technical assistance from the Duval County Health Department as part of its response to an ongoing tuberculosis (TB) outbreak among homeless persons in Florida. The request asked NIOSH to assess heating, ventilation, and air-conditioning (HVAC) systems and make recommendations to improve overall environmental controls at four homeless facilities with epidemiologic links to past or ongoing TB disease transmission.

During an on-site evaluation of the Trinity Rescue Mission homeless shelter in August 2012, we collected physical and ventilation measurements in all key areas of the facility. We focused on areas where shelter guests typically congregate or spend significant amounts of time. We recorded the make and model number of all air-handling units (AHUs) providing supply air to the facility, and visually inspected the units. When possible, we measured the air flow rate through supply diffusers and return grilles.

The ventilation systems in place could have contributed to airborne disease transmission among shelter guests. With the exception of some improper filter configurations and the use of inefficient filters in AHUs, the units typically used at the shelter appeared adequately maintained and were fully operational. Unfortunately, none of the AHUs provided fresh outdoor air to the occupied spaces, as required by the *Florida Building Code* and the American Society of Heating, Refrigerating and Air-Conditioning Engineers design standards. In addition to alleviating odors and maintaining occupant comfort, outdoor air serves to dilute infectious aerosols, such as *Mycobacterium tuberculosis* droplet nuclei that are responsible for TB transmission.

> NIOSH investigators conducted an assessment of environmental controls in the Trinity Rescue Mission, a homeless shelter linked to an ongoing tuberculosis outbreak. The investigation revealed problems with the existing environmental controls, along with needed improvements in administrative controls and respiratory protection. Detailed recommendations are provided in this report to improve the shelter environment and reduce the likelihood of disease transmission.

Since the TB outbreak began, Trinity Rescue Mission reportedly has not made any significant improvements to their administrative controls, particularly when it comes to identifying guests showing signs and symptoms of TB. We recommend that Trinity start working closely with Duval County Health Department to make improvements to the administrative controls at the shelter. From an environmental control standpoint, we suggest that all occupied spaces in the shelter are supplied adequate amounts of outdoor air based upon occupancy and room use. In addition, areas within the men's and women's facilities should be converted for use as respiratory separation areas, when necessary. These spaces could serve to separate guests suspected of having TB or other respiratory diseases from the remainder of the guest population, until medical evaluation or treatment could be obtained. To provide additional protection to the 104 guests typically housed in the men's sleeping area, we recommend installing an upper-room ultraviolet germicidal irradiation system. We also recommend developing a written infection control plan, HVAC operation and maintenance plan, and a written respiratory protection program for the shelter. Having these plans/programs in place will help Trinity Rescue Mission under normal operating conditions, and especially during future outbreaks of respiratory disease.

Keywords: NAICS 624221 (Temporary Shelters), tuberculosis, environmental controls, ventilation, homeless shelter, airborne infection, airborne transmission, respiratory

Introduction

Since 2004, the Duval County Health Department (DCHD), in conjunction with the Florida Department of Health and U.S. Centers for Disease Control and Prevention (CDC), has linked over 100 cases of active tuberculosis (TB) disease, resulting in 14 deaths, to a cluster having matching genotype results (PCR00160 or FL0046) in Duval County, Florida. Roughly half of the cases of active TB disease have been identified since 2010. Of the 100 cases, 79% had a history of homelessness, incarceration, or substance abuse, with 43% being homeless within one year of diagnosis.

In response to the ongoing outbreak, a team of epidemiologists from the CDC National Center for HIV/AIDS, Viral Hepatitis, STD, and TB Prevention (NCHHSTP), Division of Tuberculosis Elimination (DTBE) conducted an on-site investigation in February and March 2012. In their report dated April 5, 2012, the CDC team included a recommendation to improve environmental controls at homeless facilities implicated in possible disease transmission. On May 22, 2012, the Division of Respiratory Disease Studies (DRDS), National Institute for Occupational Safety and Health (NIOSH), CDC received a request for technical assistance concerning the TB outbreak in Duval County. The request was made by a CDC Public Health Advisor temporarily assigned to Duval County. The request specifically asked NIOSH to evaluate shelters' heating, ventilation, and air-conditioning (HVAC) systems and make recommendations to improve overall environmental controls. The request was initially made for an assessment at one homeless shelter. However, in subsequent discussions with the TB Program Manager at DCHD, a CDC Public Health Advisor with the Florida Department of Health, and representatives from CDC/NCHHSTP/DTBE, the request was expanded to include four facilities that provide assistance to the homeless and which had epidemiologic links to past or ongoing TB disease transmission.

In response to the expanded request, a NIOSH team visited the four facilities in August 2012. This report describes the measurements and associated findings from our assessment at the Trinity Rescue Mission. It details and prioritizes our recommendations for improving environmental controls at the shelter, and outlines the current plan for future NIOSH involvement.

Background

Tuberculosis and Homeless Populations

TB is a disease caused by *Mycobacterium tuberculosis* (*M. tuberculosis*) bacteria. When a person with active TB disease coughs or sneezes, tiny droplets containing *M. tuberculosis* may be expelled into the air. Many of these droplets dry, and the resulting residues remain suspended in the air for long periods of time as droplet nuclei. If another person inhales air that contains the infectious droplet nuclei, transmission from one person to another may occur. Homeless people have been identified as a high-risk population for TB infection and disease since the early 1900s [Knopf 1914]. With the increase in homelessness in the United States since the 1980s, TB among homeless persons has become a subject of heightened interest and concern [CDC 1985; 1992; 2003a,b; 2005a; Barry et al. 1986; Slutkin 1986; McAdam et al. 1990; Nolan 1991].

Trinity Rescue Mission

The Trinity Rescue Mission was established by the congregation of the Trinity Baptist Church to provide faith-based programs and services to homeless people in the Jacksonville community. The mission is comprised of two shelter facilities that serve the homeless year-round. The men's facility is a 12,000 square foot, single-story masonry building. Aside from a reception area and several staff offices, the building is essentially split in half by a long hallway. On one side of the hallway was a kitchen and a large open area used as a dining room and assembly space for worship services and shelter meetings. On the other side of the hallway is a large barracks-style sleeping area with an attached bathroom and shower room, laundry room, and storage areas. A total of 104 beds were available in the men's sleeping area, with 22 double bunk beds (44 total beds) located in the center of the room and 20 triple bunk beds (60 total beds) constructed along the exterior walls of the space. Four rooftop AHUs serve the spaces occupied by guests in the men's facility.

In 2006, Trinity opened a new 14,000 square foot, two-story brick Women and Children's Center to specifically meet the needs of homeless women and mothers with small children. The first floor of the facility houses a reception area, staff offices, conference room, medical clinic, dining/education area, nursery, overnight sleeping area, and six dormitory-style bedrooms, each with their own bathroom. The women's overnight sleeping area had nine bunk beds (18 total beds) for women requiring an overnight stay. The dormitory- style bedrooms were set up for between one and five guests, depending on needs. Three central AHUs located in a mechanical room provide ventilation to all occupied spaces on the first floor. The second floor of the Women and Children's Center houses 13 dormitory-style bedrooms and two larger barracks-style sleeping areas. All women living on the second floor share a large central bathroom and shower room along with a small laundry room. Four central AHUs installed in the attic provide ventilation to the occupied spaces on the second floor of the facility.

The men's facility at Trinity is usually at full capacity between men seeking overnight stays and those enrolled in the various shelter programs. When necessary, the dining/assembly area can be used to house men in excess of the 104 available beds. The Women and Children's Center had the capacity to house 100 guests or more, but only 50-60 guests reside there on average.

Assessment

On August 20, 2012, an opening meeting was held at the Duval County Health Department. An update was given on the current status of the ongoing TB outbreak among the homeless population, and we provided background information on NIOSH, the nature of the technical assistance request, and the ventilation measurements we planned to collect at each facility. Aside from NIOSH and DCHD staff, representatives from three other homeless facilities to be visited during the week were in attendance. There was not a representative from Trinity Rescue Mission present at the meeting.

We arrived at Trinity Rescue Mission on Thursday, August 23, 2012, and met briefly with the Director of Operations. After we unloaded our ventilation equipment, a member of the maintenance staff provided a tour of the men's facility and led us across the parking lot to the Women and Children's Center. While there, staff members provided a tour of both floors, and we began taking physical and ventilation measurements in all key areas of the facility. We focused on areas where Trinity guests typically congregate or spend significant amounts of time.

We recorded the make and model number of all nine air-handling units (AHUs) providing supply air to the two buildings, and we visually inspected all of the units. When possible, we measured the air flow rate through supply diffusers and return grilles using a TSI Incorporated (Shoreview, Minnesota) Model 8373 Accubalance Plus equipped with air capture hood appropriately sized to accommodate each supply diffuser and return grille. The Model 8373 measures volumetric air flow rates of 30–2000 cubic feet per minute (cfm) with an accuracy of ±5% of the reading and ±5 cfm. The Accubalance Plus is also equipped with a directional air flow indicator that provides confirmation of flow direction. We determined the approximate internal volume of the measured spaces with either a standard tape measure or a Zircon Corporation (Campbell, California) Model 58026 LaserVision DM200 laser distance measuring device. The device accurately measures up to 200 feet and has function keys for calculating the area and volume of a room for HVAC load formulas. When the existence of air flow or the air flow direction was questioned, we used a Wizard Stick hand-held fog generator (Zero Toys, Concord, Massachusetts) to confirm and visualize the air flow pattern.

After recording our measurements, we intended to meet briefly with the Trinity Director of Operations to discuss our general findings. However, he was out of the office and unavailable at the time, so a meeting did not occur. A formal closing meeting for our on-site response to the technical assistance request for all four facilities was held on August 23, 2012, at the DCHD. This meeting provided us an opportunity to discuss our general findings with representatives from the Duval County Health Department. There was not a representative from Trinity Rescue Mission present at the meeting.

Results and Discussion

General Tuberculosis Infection Control

All tuberculosis control programs should include three key components: administrative controls (e.g., intake questionnaires and policies), environmental controls (e.g., ventilation and filtration), and a respiratory protection program. Ideally, environmental controls and respiratory protection should supplement aggressive administrative controls. Detailed explanations for each of these key control elements, as well as a discussion on the hierarchy of their implementation, are outlined in CDC's *Guidelines for Preventing the Transmission of* Mycobacterium tuberculosis *in Health-Care Settings, 2005* and P*revention and Control of Tuberculosis in Correctional and Detention Facilities: Recommendations from CDC* [CDC 2005b, 2006]. In high risk environments, such as homeless shelters, or in areas where administrative controls alone are inadequate, environmental controls and respiratory protection should be used as secondary and tertiary levels of control, respectively.

Administrative Controls

Limited administrative controls for preventing the transmission of airborne diseases were in place at the shelter prior to the current disease outbreak. Shelter staff confirmed this fact during our visit, and staff members also reported that Trinity had not implemented any new administrative procedures or policies in response to the ongoing outbreak. Unlike many other homeless facilities in the area, we also learned that Trinity elected not to participate in response efforts by DCHD or the Jacksonville Community Tuberculosis Coalition.

As with most homeless facilities, Trinity frequently provides services to large numbers of guests in close proximity to one another. This is particularly the case in the congregate sleeping areas and dining/assembly areas in the men's and women's facilities. Even the best ventilation systems are incapable of preventing the spread of disease between guests close to one another. Thus, establishing policies and procedures to rapidly identify people with suspected disease, keep them separated from the general guest population, and follow up with appropriate medical evaluations and treatment (if necessary) is the most important element in reducing or eliminating the spread of disease. We recommend taking steps to train employees and volunteers on symptoms of TB disease and the prevention of TB transmission. Additionally, screening procedures should be developed and implemented to help identify guests on target screening lists, or others suspected of having TB. These guests should then be referred to DCHD for critical medical testing and care. While enhanced training and detailed administrative policies would help identify guests at risk for disease during the current TB outbreak, having new controls in place would reduce the likelihood of airborne disease transmission at the shelter in the future as well.

While taking critical steps to enhance the administrative controls at Trinity would be a significant step, the development of a written TB Infection Control Plan (ICP) for the shelter is strongly recommended. At the time of the NIOSH investigation, no such ICP was reported to exist. Information on creating detailed ICPs and TB ICP templates for homeless shelters can be found at the Curry International Tuberculosis Center website at http://www.currytbcenter. ucsf.edu/. Collaborating with DCHD and the Florida Department of Health would serve to further strengthen the written plan. These ICPs are particularly useful when overall TB infection control requires the coordination and subsequent follow-up of different agencies. For an ICP to be effective, the process should be formally documented in a protocol or checklist format. This ensures that each time there is a TB-related incident, all necessary agencies understand their responsibilities and perform their necessary predetermined actions in a consistent manner. Incorporating the input of staff involved in the maintenance and operation of facility ventilation systems into the overall infection control program strengthens the program and provides these staff members with additional insight as to what ventilation requirements are necessary to prevent and/or isolate TB disease. Input from the ventilation staff should be sought during the formal creation of the ICP and during subsequent revisions to the plan.

Environmental Controls
General Ventilation System Information

General information on the AHUs at Trinity, including the areas served by each unit, is provided in Table 1. Of the 11 total AHUs, 10 of the units were produced by Carrier Corporation (Farmington, Connecticut). AHU Men-3 was produced by Goodman Manufacturing (Houston, Texas). The four AHUs serving the guest areas of the men's facility are mounted on the roof of the men's facility. In the women's facility, three AHUs provide ventilation for the first floor of the building. Those units are all located in a large mechanical room on the first floor of the Women and Children's Center. Four additional AHUs are mounted in the attic of the women's facility to provide ventilation to the living areas on the second floor of the building. All 11 AHUs supply air to occupied spaces through galvanized steel and flexible fiberglass supply ducts. The return air flows back to the units through ducted returns or ceiling plenums. None of the AHUs delivered fresh outdoor air into the buildings.

On the day of our visit, AHU Men-1, AHU Men-2, and AHU Men-4 on the roof of the men's facility were operational and capable of maintaining temperature set points and air flow. It was reported that AHU Men-4, serving the men's kitchen, is rarely used. This was confirmed by the cleanliness of the filters inside that unit when compared to filters in the others. During our visit, AHU Men-4 was not powered on, so we could not confirm the operational status of the unit. The seven AHUs in the Women and Children's Center were fairly new, and they were all operational and capable of maintaining temperature set points and air flow. The mechanical room housing the three AHUs on the first floor of the women's facility was clean and free of clutter, which allowed unfettered access to the three units. The four units in the attic were easily accessible via a wooden walkway constructed in the attic space.

Filtration

As shown in Figure 1, AHU Men-1, AHU Men-2, and AHU Men-4 had ventilation filters that appeared to be homemade and not commercially-available. Each of the AHUs had four of the homemade filters inside. While the manufacturer prescribes four filters installed in each unit, the size of the homemade filters did not match the prescribed filter size. While the homemade filters provided some level of filtration, the level of efficiency was uncertain as the deviation from intended design provided ample opportunity for filter failure and bypass. AHU Men-3 contained a set of four properly-sized disposable panel filters from Glasfloss Industries (Dallas, Texas). The Glasfloss disposable panel filters do not have a published American Society of Heating, Refrigerating and Air-Conditioning Engineers (ASHRAE) Minimum Efficiency Reporting Value (MERV), which relates to filtration efficiency. However, disposable panel filters typically fall into a MERV range of 4 to 6, which corresponds to a removal efficiency of up to 50% for 3.0 to 10 micrometer (μm) particles [ANSI/ASHRAE 2007]. However, MERV 4-6 filters are less than 20% efficient at filtering particles in the 1.0–3.0 μm size range, which includes droplet nuclei responsible for *M. tuberculosis* transmission [ANSI/ASHRAE 2007]. All of the ventilation filters used in the Women and Children's Center were Flanders Corporation (Washington, North Carolina) EZ-Flow disposable panel filters. The EZFlow filters have an established ASHRAE MERV of 4, so their efficiency is likely comparable to the disposable panel filters described above.

To prevent the spread of *M. tuberculosis*, air filters should provide a removal efficiency of greater than 90% of particles in the 1.0–3.0 μm size range (corresponding to a MERV 13 or higher). During any future HVAC design modifications, system evaluations, or retrofits, the selection of filters for use in the AHUs, especially those serving the three main overnight sleeping areas, should be closely examined. Care should be taken when choosing more efficient filters, because increased efficiency is typically associated with increased pressure drop across the filter (resistance to air flow). Filters in the AHUs should have the highest possible efficiency (i.e., highest MERV rating) while still maintaining the air flow required for conditioning and outdoor air supply through each system.

Preventive Maintenance

The ventilation system preventive maintenance program at Trinity was coordinated by shelter administrators. With the exception of the homemade and low-efficiency filter issues, all of the AHUs were clean and appeared to be adequately maintained. We were unable to determine the frequency of ventilation filter replacement. Unfortunately, there is no written plan outlining the preventive maintenance schedules and procedures for the shelter HVAC systems. A written HVAC Operation and Maintenance (O&M) Plan should be developed. Combining all maintenance tasks, schedules, procedures, and training requirements into a written plan would help ensure that all equipment is properly maintained at appropriate time intervals and that any emergency maintenance issues are addressed correctly. Consultation with the filter media manufacturer or their vendor representative(s) should provide the recommended filter replacement frequency for inclusion into the O&M plan. A detailed plan would also help ensure that the quality of work remains consistent as staff changes. Once developed, this written plan should be revised periodically to be current with any ventilation system and equipment modifications at the facility.

Ventilation Measurements and Indoor Air Quality

An adequate supply of outdoor air, typically delivered through the HVAC system, is necessary in any indoor environment to dilute pollutants that are released by equipment, building materials, furnishings, products, and people. In the State of Florida, the 2010 *Florida Building Code* mandates "minimum requirements to safeguard the public health, safety and general welfare through structural strength, means of egress facilities, stability, sanitation, adequate light and ventilation, energy conservation, and safety to life and property from fire and other hazards attributed to the built environment and to provide safety to fire fighters and emergency responders during emergency operations [ICC 2011]." The *Florida Building Code* applies to the "construction, alteration, movement, enlargement, replacement, repair, equipment, use and occupancy, location, maintenance, removal and demolition of every building or structure or any appurtenances connected or attached to such buildings or structures" throughout the state. The Code is based on a variety of model building codes and consensus standards from national organizations, which have been modified to fit Florida's specific needs, when necessary. When it comes to ventilation standards, in most cases, the *Florida Building Code* has adopted the recommendations published in *American National Standards Institute (ANSI)/ASHRAE Standard 62.1-2010: Ventilation for Acceptable Indoor Air Quality*. These ASHRAE recommendations provide specific details on ventilation for acceptable indoor air quality [ANSI/ASHRAE 2010a].

The 2010 *Florida Building Code* and ASHRAE 62.1-2010 recommend outdoor air supply rates that take into account people-related contaminant sources as well as building-related contaminant sources. Similarly, exhaust air flow rate requirements for some spaces are also listed. Although there are no specific guidelines for homeless shelters and related facilities, there are published guidelines applicable to Trinity. These outdoor air supply and exhaust air requirements are summarized in Table 2. Table 2 also lists the default occupant densities for various spaces. These default values, given in terms of number of occupants per 1000 square feet, are provided by the *Florida Building Code* and ASHRAE to assist building and HVAC system designers when actual occupant densities are unknown. Although actual occupant densities for the occupied spaces of the shelter are generally known, the default values still serve as a reference to determine whether the occupant density in a given space is higher or lower than what is considered typical.

The physical and ventilation measurements we collected are presented in Table 3. The second-to-last column of the table presents the actual occupant densities in each space. Values preceded by an asterisk (*) denote areas with occupant densities above typical values (i.e., higher than the default values presented in Table 2). High occupant densities are not solely indicative of ventilation problems. However, the men's sleeping area and the women's overnight sleeping room show high occupant densities because many people actually sleep in close proximity to one another. Some of the women's rooms on the first floor of the Women and Children's Center could have high occupant densities when they are filled to their reported capacities. In these cases, special consideration should be given to air flow patterns in the spaces to minimize the potential of exhalations from one person passing through the breathing zone of multiple other people. This is especially true when airborne disease transmission is a concern.

The last column in Table 3 presents the outdoor air requirements for each space, as established by the 2010 *Florida Building Code* and ASHRAE. As previously noted, none of the AHUs at Trinity were delivering any fresh outdoor air into the building. While the rooftop AHUs on the men's facility could easily be modified to bring in outdoor air, the AHUs in the women's facility were not installed in a way that would allow them to easily bring outdoor air into the building. Before modifying any of the AHUs to bring in outdoor air, it needs to be determined whether each individual AHU has the tempering capacity to incorporate the introduction of outdoor air. If such capacity is available, introducing outdoor air through the AHUs would require some modifications and result in increased annual energy costs. However, it is important to ensure that all occupied spaces in Trinity are receiving adequate amounts of fresh outdoor air to inhibit airborne disease transmission and improve indoor air quality. In addition to alleviating odors and better maintaining occupant comfort, outdoor air serves to dilute infectious aerosols, such as *M. tuberculosis* droplet nuclei.

Two common approaches could be employed by Trinity to introduce outdoor air into the occupied spaces (or a combination of the two). The first approach would be to make the necessary modifications to the existing AHUs to allow them to bring in the required outdoor air. This would initially require evaluation, by a knowledgeable HVAC engineer (a reputable ventilation or engineering design contractor that is familiar with ASHRAE, Facility Guidelines Institute [FGI], and CDC guidelines and recommendations), of each AHU's conditioning capacity to determine if it can handle the additional tempering and dehumidification burden introduced by the outdoor air. Assuming that such conditioning capacity exists, modifying the AHUs on the roof of the men's facility should be made easier by the fact that these units are already located outdoors. The system modifications for the AHUs in the women's facility would require more extensive modifications since the required outdoor air intakes and dampers would need to be installed into the spaces housing these AHUs. Although incorporating outdoor air into the existing AHUs may be the simpler of the two solutions and could require the least capital expense, it may cost significantly more in energy over time. In their current configurations, the AHUs are simply recirculating air that is relatively close to the desired indoor temperature and humidity conditions. After circulating through the occupied space, this air requires less conditioning to return it to the desired delivery temperature and humidity levels. Once outdoor air is mixed in with the room return air, the mixed air stream introduced to each AHU will be further from the desired indoor conditions for most of the year. Each AHU will then need to work harder to dehumidify and temper the mixed air stream.

A second common method of bringing outdoor air into the shelter would be to install a dedicated outdoor air system. This would involve installing a completely new AHU for the men's facility, with ductwork extending to all occupied spaces of the building. A separate dedicated outdoor air system would similarly be required for the women's facility. For the men's building, the new AHU should be sized to provide adequate outdoor air flow for the entire building (approximately 1600 to 1800 cfm) while also providing the entire capacity to temper and dehumidify this outdoor air. Similarly, the new AHU for the women's facility would need to provide around 1500 cfm of outdoor air. The new AHUs should provide tempered and dehumidified (supercooled to 45–50°F dew point) outdoor air to each space (or existing AHU) in quantities necessary to meet *Florida Building Code* and ASHRAE outdoor air requirements. Terminal reheating or blending of this air with air delivered by the primary AHUs may be necessary to prevent thermal discomfort from the supercooled outdoor air. Conversely, multiple smaller dedicated outdoor air systems could serve the same purpose as one large system for the entire main building. Regardless of how it is accomplished, the primary advantage of the dedicated outdoor air system is that it would not require major modifications to the existing AHUs, which would simply continue to recirculate air through the spaces they serve while providing air filtration, heating and cooling. The dedicated outdoor air system would certainly require more capital expense and more renovations for the required ductwork than the first option, but it could also provide significant energy cost savings, making it a more viable long-term solution.

A knowledgeable HVAC engineer should be consulted to discuss these and other potential options for introducing outdoor air into the shelters. At the same time, consideration should be given to optimizing air flow patterns, particularly in the men's sleeping area and the women's overnight sleeping room, to reduce the potential of airborne disease transmission between guests. While even the best ventilation system cannot guarantee prevention of disease transmission between people in close proximity to one another, improving air flow patterns could help reduce the overall transmission potential among guests in each sleeping area. One way that air flow patterns could be improved in these areas is to supply all air (fresh and recirculated) above the center aisles between rows of beds using supply diffusers designed to discharge the air in a wide, downward deflected angle. At the same time, return grills should be installed along the perimeter of each space. In this arrangement, supply air will generally pass over/across each bed and directly back to the AHU. This will reduce the potential of exhalations from one person passing through the breathing zone of multiple other people sharing the space. This arrangement should also alleviate concerns with short-circuiting of air, where supply air is immediately pulled into a return grille without providing any useful ventilation. Short-circuiting of air is a special concern in the men's sleeping area since all of the supply vents and return grilles are currently located in only one wall of the room. Luckily, the 15-feet ceiling height in the men's sleeping area would allow for easier implementation of ventilation improvements than would otherwise be the case. A qualified HVAC/ventilation engineer might recommend other air flow schemes that could be similarly effective at providing adequate ventilation while minimizing the potential for disease transmission. The final chosen design scheme should be qualitatively smoke/fog tested to verify performance.

During our visit, we collected measurements in the clinic area on the first floor of the Women and Children's Center and identified two separate examination rooms. Our measurements show (see Table 3), and ventilation fog testing confirmed, that exam room #1 and possibly exam room #2 (the return grille was obstructed) were improperly maintained under positive pressure compared to the adjacent waiting area. Thus, air from inside an exam room migrates out of the space into the waiting area. Any areas used for medical evaluations should be maintained under negative pressure relative to the surrounding areas, and the pressure relationship should be periodically tested and confirmed with a micromanometer or visual techniques like smoke tubes or flutter strips. Thus, ventilation changes should be made to create a proper air flow pattern that helps keep any airborne infectious agents generated inside an exam room from traveling to the adjacent waiting area. The correct negative pressure could possibly be established by adjusting existing dampers or ductwork so more air is exhausted from the exam rooms than is being supplied to them. Reducing return air from adjacent rooms on the same HVAC system will facilitate this approach. If negative pressure cannot be maintained with such adjustments, the installation of dedicated exhaust fans within each exam room may be required. Depending upon frequency of patient exams, the dedicated exhaust fan approach could be a more energy-efficient option for maintaining negative pressure in these areas, though administrative or occupancy-automated procedures to ensure their use during patient exams would be of primary importance.

We also noticed that none of the exhaust fans from bathrooms on the first floor of the women's facility were functioning properly during our visit (see Table 3). To control humidity and odors, bathrooms and shower areas should exhaust more air than the AHU is supplying. This will maintain these areas under negative pressure. Separate exhaust fans should be used to exhaust air directly outside at least 25 feet from any air intakes. There should be no recycling or re-entrainment of return/exhaust air from the bathrooms and shower rooms. For high occupancy public bathrooms, 50 cfm of exhaust per toilet/urinal is recommended. For private toilets in bathrooms intended to be occupied by only one person at a time, ASHRAE 62.1-2010 specifies that the exhaust ventilation should be 25 cfm if the exhaust fan is designed to operate continuously (the *Florida Building Code* only requires 20 cfm) or 50 cfm if the exhaust fan only operates during periods of occupancy (e.g., exhaust fan controlled by a wall switch). The bathroom exhaust fans should be made functional with their exhaust rates verified for compliance with the 2010 *Florida Building Code*, and they should be operational any time the bathrooms are occupied. [Note: The kitchen hood exhaust systems were not evaluated at the time of the NIOSH site visit. These systems are not discussed in this report.]

While not a major concern from an airborne disease transmission standpoint, temperature and relative humidity (RH) affect the perception of comfort in an indoor environment. The perception of thermal comfort is related to one's metabolic heat production, the transfer of heat to the environment, physiological adjustments, and body temperature. Heat transfer from the body to the environment is influenced by factors such as temperature, humidity, air movement, personal activities, and clothing. *ANSI/ASHRAE Standard 55-2010: Thermal Environmental Conditions for Human Occupancy* specifies conditions in which 80% or more of the occupants are expected to find the environment thermally acceptable [ANSI/ASHRAE 2010b]. Assuming slow air movement and 50% RH, the operative temperatures recommended by ASHRAE range from 68.5°F–76°F in the winter, and from 75.5°F–80.5°F in the summer (see Table 4). The difference between the two temperature ranges is largely due to seasonal clothing selection. ASHRAE also recommends that RH be maintained at or below 65%. The U.S. Environmental Protection Agency recommends maintaining indoor relative humidity between 30–50% because excessive humidity can promote the growth of microorganisms [EPA 2012]. Temperature and RH levels were not recorded during our visit because the main guest spaces were generally empty. We recommend maintaining the indoor temperature and RH levels within the ranges established by ASHRAE to provide the most comfortable environment to guests at Trinity. Meeting the 30–50% RH recommendation would be significantly easier if a dedicated outdoor air system is installed to introduce conditioned outdoor air to the shelter, as explained above.

Respiratory Separation Areas

Currently, Trinity does not have areas set aside for separating guests suspected of having TB or other respiratory diseases from the remainder of the guest population. Rapidly identifying people with suspected TB disease and keeping them separated from others until appropriate medical evaluations and treatments are initiated is one of the most important elements in reducing or eliminating the spread of airborne disease. Since the backgrounds and medical statuses may be unknown for overnight guests, we strongly recommend identifying separate areas in the men's and women's shelters, which can be used for respiratory separation when needed. It is important to recognize that respiratory separation is not an alternative to medical evaluation. Rather, it is proposed to be a temporary holding area for guests awaiting transport for medical evaluation. It may also be used to house guests exhibiting signs of respiratory distress without having identified disease. When respiratory separation is not required, the areas can be used for normal guest housing or other purposes.

A respiratory separation area is not intended to be equivalent to an airborne infection isolation (AII) patient room found in hospitals and other healthcare settings. However, it can be designed using some of the same protective concepts, namely negative room pressure and elevated ventilation rates. The respiratory separation area should be maintained under negative pressure relative to the adjacent spaces. This means that air from outside the respiratory separation area should migrate inwards into the respiratory separation area and not in the opposite direction. This is easily maintained by exhausting more air from the respiratory separation area than is being supplied. Operable windows, either within the respiratory separation area or in adjacent areas, should not be allowed to interfere with this intent. Negative pressure helps reduce the potential that any guest housed in the respiratory separation area with active TB disease (or any other disease where airborne infection is a concern) could expose other healthy individuals in adjacent areas. In addition to maintaining negative pressure, all return air from the respiratory separation area should preferably be exhausted directly outside. In no circumstances should air from the respiratory separation area be allowed to re-infiltrate the building or go back through the AHU without first having passed through a high-efficiency particulate air (HEPA) filter.

For true AII rooms in healthcare facilities, the CDC and FGI recommend a differential pressure of ≥ 0.01 inches of water gauge (2.5 Pascals [Pa]) across the closed door between the isolation area and adjacent areas [CDC 2005b; FGI 2010]. Although the minimum pressure difference needed for maintaining airflow into a room is quite small (about 0.001 inches of water gauge), the higher prescribed pressure differential is easier to measure and maintain as the pressure in surrounding areas changes due to the opening and closing of doors, ventilation system fluctuations, and other factors. The FGI and CDC also recommend a total of 12 air changes per hour (ACH) through the isolation room (CDC allows 6 ACH for existing AII rooms) and at least 2 ACH of fresh outdoor air. True AII rooms are designed to house individuals with confirmed respiratory disease. A respiratory separation area at Trinity would not be used to house guests with confirmed disease, so it would not be necessary to meet the strict air flow and differential pressure requirements detailed above. However, knowledge of the AII design strategies could be useful in designing a respiratory separation area. It is vastly more important to establish a negative pressure area that can be used for respiratory separation than it is to focus on the respiratory separation area meeting quantitative ventilation requirements.

During our visit, we noticed that rooms 1-6 on the first floor of the women's facility as areas that could effectively be converted to respiratory separation areas. At least one of these small housing rooms should be upgraded to serve this purpose. One or more of these rooms could be converted for respiratory separation by 1) installing a solid, sealed ceiling in place of the existing drop ceiling or ensuring the walls for the selected room extend to the hard ceiling above the current drop ceiling, 2) installing a new dedicated exhaust fan through the outside wall of each selected room to provide the required exhaust air flow when the room was in use for respiratory separation, and 3) installing tight-closing dampers (or some other mechanism) to completely seal all existing air returns from each selected room (including the bathroom) to the AHU serving the room. An exhaust fan should be chosen that is capable of maintaining the room under negative pressure relative to the adjacent corridor with minimal noise. These fans could be mounted directly in the wall or on the roof with ductwork running through the wall and up to the fans on the outside of the shelter. Placement of the fan intakes within the room's private bathroom itself may be required in order to maintain the restroom at negative pressure relative to the sleeping area. It is imperative that exhaust air from these new fans is directed away from all future AHU air intakes and gathering areas outside the shelter.

For the rooms selected for respiratory separation and when respiratory separation is desired, the newly installed return air dampers should be sealed to prevent air from inside the room returning to the AHU. The new exhaust fan should also be activated to maintain the space under negative pressure. For the majority of the time, when respiratory separation is not required, the room can be used as normal by deactivating the exhaust fan and reopening the return air dampers back to the AHU.

Aside from staff offices, there were no areas identified in the men's shelter that could readily be converted into a space for respiratory separation. Since all men staying at the shelter sleep in the same large barracks-style sleeping area, ideally a small room should be constructed in a corner of the sleeping area specifically for respiratory separation. Having a separate room would allow the space to be used for separation purposes by following the same procedures outlined above for spaces in the women's shelter (except there may not be a return air grille that needs sealed). If construction of a separate room is impractical, an alternative (but less-desirable) approach is to install impervious retractable partitions (e.g. accordion-type room dividers) that could be used to enclose a corner of the men's sleeping area when respiratory separation is warranted. The partitions should touch the floor and extend as close to the roof deck as possible. An exhaust fan would need to be installed through one of the solid walls enclosed by the partitions. Again, the fan could be mounted directly in the wall or on the roof with ductwork running through the wall and up to the fan on the outside of the shelter. It is imperative that exhaust air from this new fan is directed away from all future AHU air intakes and gathering areas outside the shelter. Since there would be more leakage into the separation area around the partition walls, a larger fan would likely be required to maintain negative pressure over that required for a solid room.

If a retractable partition enclosure is selected for respiratory separation in the men's shelter, the partitions should fit as snug to the floor and ceiling as possible. The new exhaust fan should also be activated to maintain the enclosed space under negative pressure. For the majority of the time, when respiratory separation is not required, the corner of the room can be used as normal by shutting down the exhaust fan and pushing the retractable partitions out of the way.

For any respiratory separation area, a written plan for testing and operating the space is strongly recommended. At Trinity, a detailed written plan should be developed for the rapid conversion of the spaces from standard housing areas to use for respiratory separation. The plan should include contingency plans for moving the guests currently housed in the spaces to other locations, steps for cleaning and refurnishing the areas for separation purposes, and step-by-step procedures for shelter staff to follow to effectively initiate respiratory separation.

When occupied for separation purposes, all respiratory separation areas should be visually tested daily to ensure negative pressure is being maintained. Testing can be done cheaply and easily with tissue flutter strips or smoke tubes. The results of the testing should be documented each day when in use. When the spaces are being used for normal guest housing, they should be tested a minimum of once per month to ensure proper operation in the event they would be needed for respiratory separation.

Auxiliary HEPA Filtration
The higher the dilution ventilation rate within a given respiratory separation area, the faster the room air will be cleared of existing airborne pathogens. In order to increase effective ventilation within a separation area, in-room HEPA filtration units may be used. These units may be portable or permanently-mounted somewhere within the space. Some models can be ceiling mounted, which could reduce the potential for tampering. If such units are used, their placement and discharge orientation must be selected, installed, and maintained carefully to maximize room air mixing effectiveness without disrupting the desired flow of air into the respiratory separation area. These criteria become even more important if a retractable partition enclosure is used to establish a respiratory separation area.

One unique use of portable HEPA filtration units is through the use of a *ventilated headboard*. The ventilated headboard is a NIOSH-developed technology that consists of lightweight, sturdy & adjustable aluminum framing with a retractable plastic canopy sheeting that can extend over the pillow area of a cot, mat or bed. Low-velocity airflow into the canopy is created using a high-efficiency fan/filter exhaust unit. This local control technique allows for near-instant capture of any aerosol originating from the patient while simultaneously providing air cleaning to the entire room. NIOSH engineers are available to provide additional information or to assist in the selection and acquisition of ventilated headboards.

Ultraviolet Germicidal Irradiation
Ultraviolet germicidal irradiation (UVGI) is the use of ultraviolet (UV) energy (electromagnetic radiation with a wavelength shorter than that of visible light) to kill or inactivate viral, bacterial, and fungal organisms. The UV spectrum is commonly divided into UVA (wavelengths of 400-315 nm), UVB (315-280 nm), and UVC (280-200 nm). The entire UV spectrum can kill or inactivate microorganisms, but UVC energy provides the most germicidal effect, with 265 nm being the optimum wavelength [ASHRAE 2011, 2012]. Modern UV lamps primarily create UVC energy at a near-optimal 254 nm by electrical discharge through low-pressure gas (including mercury vapor) enclosed in a quartz tube. UVC from mercury lamps is often referred to as UVGI to denote its germicidal properties. Although UVC is invisible to the human eye, small amounts of energy released at visible

wavelengths produce the blue glow commonly associated with UVC lamps.

Research has demonstrated that UVGI is effective in killing or inactivating *M. tuberculosis* under experimental conditions [Riley et al. 1957, 1962; Riley and Nardell 1989; Xu et al. 2003]. UVGI has also proven effective in reducing the transmission of other infectious agents in hospitals, military housing units, and class rooms [Willmon et al. 1948; Wells and Holla 1950; McLean 1961]. Due to the results of controlled studies and the experiences of clinicians and engineers, UVGI has been recommended as a supplement to other TB infection-control and ventilation measures to kill or inactivate *M. tuberculosis* [David 1973; Riley et al. 1976; CDC 2005b, NIOSH 2009].

In congregate settings typical in homeless shelters and healthcare facilities, upper-room UVGI systems (often called upper-air systems) are often used to interrupt the transmission of airborne infectious pathogens within the occupied spaces themselves. Upper-room UV lamp fixtures are suspended from the ceiling and/or mounted on walls at a minimum height of 7 feet above the floor (Figure 2) [Riley and Nardell 1989; Brickner et al. 2003; NIOSH 2009; ASHRAE 2011, 2012]. Lamps are shielded to direct radiation upward and outward to create an intense zone of UVC in the upper portion of the room while minimizing UVC levels in the lower occupied spaces. These fixtures inactivate airborne microorganisms by irradiating them as air currents move them into the path of the UV energy. Some upper-room lamp fixtures utilize small fans to enhance air mixing (right photograph in Figure 2) [First et al. 1999a,b; CDC 2005b; NIOSH 2009; ASHRAE 2011, 2012]. The overall effectiveness of upper-room UVGI systems improves significantly when the space is well mixed [Riley and Nardell 1989; Brickner et al. 2003]. Although convection air currents created by occupants and equipment can provide adequate air circulation in some settings, mechanical ventilation systems and/or ceiling fans that maximize air mixing are preferable. Floor fans can also be placed in the room to ensure adequate mixing.

Application and placement criteria for upper- room UV fixtures are provided in various publications, and manufacturer-specific advice on placement and operations should always be followed [First et al. 1999a,b; Riley and Nardell 1989; Brickner et al. 2003; CDC 2005b; NIOSH 2009; ASHRAE 2011, 2012]. For decades, a rule of thumb for upper-air installations has been one 30-watt (nominal input) fixture for every 200 square feet of floor space to be irradiated [Riley and Nardell 1989]. Many effective systems have been designed to this criterion, yet it is important to note that not all 30-watt lamps provide the same output of UVC energy. Ultimately, UVC output is dependent on the type of lamp, the lamp manufacturer, the ballast used to power the lamp, the complete fixture design, and many other factors. A more recent study has suggested installing fixtures to maintain a uniform UV distribution of around 30-50 microwatts of UVC energy per square centimeter (μW/cm^2) in the upper portion of the room [Xu et al. 2003]. While essentially "normalizing" the recommended output over all lamps and fixture designs, this level of irradiance should be effective at inactivating most airborne droplet nuclei containing Mycobacterium, and would presumably be effective for inactivation of most viruses as well. Using the results of the Xu et al. study, NIOSH developed guidelines for designing upper-room UVGI systems for controlling the spread of tuberculosis [NIOSH 2009]. While the guidelines were specifically targeted for healthcare settings, they are just as applicable to congregate sleeping areas in homeless facilities.

We recommend consulting with a qualified UVGI fixture manufacturer or system engineer, familiar with the NIOSH upper-room UVGI guidelines, to design and install an upper-air UVGI system in the men's sleeping area at Trinity. The 15-feet ceiling height in that space provides an excellent opportunity to utilize a variety of commercially-available fixtures to create a large irradiance zone in the upper portion of the room. The ability to mount the fixtures at higher heights will also help prevent the fixtures from being tampered with. The system should be designed to provide UV irradiance levels of at least 30-50 μW/cm^2 in the upper portion of the room while limiting UVC exposure to occupants in the space, particularly men sleeping or sitting on top bunk beds. If desired, NIOSH engineers are available to review any proposed UVGI design strategies prior to their purchase and installation.

In humans, UVGI may be absorbed by the outer surfaces of the eyes and skin. Short-term overexposure may result in photokeratitis (inflammation of the cornea) and/or keratoconjunctivitis (inflammation of the conjunctiva). The NIOSH Recommended Exposure Limit (REL) for ultraviolet irradiation (254 nm) is 6.0 millijoules per square centimeter (mJ/cm^2) for an 8-hour exposure time [NIOSH 1972; ACGIH 2012]. This REL corresponds to a maximum continuous exposure of 0.2 μW/cm^2 of irradiation to a person inside the room over the 8-hour period. If periods of longer potential exposures are anticipated, the measured UV irradiance in the lower portion of the room should be lower than 0.2 μW/cm^2. The NIOSH guidelines clearly explain calculating permissible exposure times given actual irradiance levels in the occupied zone. Actual UVC irradiance levels in the occupied portion of the room, along with corresponding permissible exposure times, should be measured and documented by the system designer/installer prior to initial system use.

Once the upper-room UVGI system is in place and working properly, the fixtures should be operated any time occupants are in the men's sleeping area. It is preferable to operate the system 24 hours per day every day. As with any environmental control system, the new upper-room UVGI system will require periodic maintenance. The output from UV lamps naturally decreases over time as the lamps are burned. Frequently turning the lamps off and on also shortens the useful life of the lamps. The UV output from lamps will also decrease due to accumulated dust. Therefore, lamps should be inspected periodically (e.g., quarterly) and cleaned when necessary. UV lamps are typically cleaned by wiping the lamp tubes with isopropyl alcohol (rubbing alcohol) and a clean, lint-free cloth. Cleaning the lamps with water can result in smearing of the dust that can further reduce lamp performance. The fixtures housing the UV lamps should be inspected and cleaned as well. Typical UVGI lamps are rated for around a year of continuous use. Lamps should be replaced annually, or in accordance with appropriate manufacturer recommendations.

IMPORTANT SAFETY PRECAUTION: All UVGI systems must be inactivated before workers enter the upper irradiated upper portion of the space. All Trinity personnel that might spend time in the men's sleeping area should be trained in exposure hazards posed by the UVGI fixtures. Employees responsible for lamp and fixture maintenance should receive additional safety training. All initial maintenance and training requirements should be explained by the UVGI system designer/installer. The required maintenance tasks and service logs, along with training requirements and logs should be included in the written O&M plan recommended above. A subcomponent of this plan should include a UVGI safety plan. Complete information on upper-room UVGI system design, operation, maintenance, and safety can be found in the NIOSH guideline document available online at: http://www.cdc.gov/niosh/docs/2009-105/pdfs/2009-105.pdf [NIOSH 2009].

Respiratory Protection

During an outbreak of airborne infectious disease, there could be instances when staff members find themselves in close contact with guests suspected of being infectious. One example would be a van driver transporting clients to/from Community Rehabilitation Center. Ideally, these cases would be identified during the administrative screening process. When these circumstances cannot be avoided, it is wise to consider the availability of respiratory protection to protect staff members. The first step toward the implementation of respirator use is to develop a document that clearly outlines a formal respiratory protection program. The Occupational Safety and Health Administration (OSHA) Respiratory Protection standard (29 Code of Federal Regulations [CFR] 1910.134) outlines the requirements for comprehensive respiratory protection programs. In accordance with 29 CFR 1910.134, a written Respiratory Protection Program, with an identified program administrator, is required for any facility that requires employees to wear respirators. The program must include training, medical evaluations, and respirators at no cost to employees or staff required to wear respirators on the job. Initial fit testing by a trained individual is required for all employees that will potentially wear a respirator. Annual fit testing is required after that, with additional fit testing upon major changes to the facial features of the respirator user (i.e. major weight gain/loss, change in facial hair, scarring, etc.).

To comply with applicable OSHA regulations regarding respiratory protection, we recommend that Community Rehabilitation Center create a written respiratory protection program as outlined in 29 CFR 1910.134, appoint a program administrator, and initiate training and initial fit testing for employees. Many online resources exist to assist in the development of a respiratory protection program. OSHA has published a Respiratory Protection informational booklet online (http://www.osha.gov/Publications/OSHA3079/osha3079.html) and a more detailed Small Entity Compliance Guide for the Revised Respiratory Protection Standard (http://www.osha.gov/Publications/3384small-entity-for-respiratory-protection-standard-rev.pdf) to explain all parts of an appropriate respiratory protection program and how to comply. The Small Entity Compliance Guide also contains a sample respiratory protection program in Attachment 4 that can be used as a model program. The Washington State Department of Labor and Industries has also developed a user-friendly, fillable template that is helpful in developing a respiratory protection program at http://www.lni.wa.gov/Safety/Basics/Programs/Accident/Samples/RespProtectguide2.doc.

The DCHD, Florida Department of Health, local healthcare facilities or fire/ambulance stations can potentially assist with training and fit testing the employees required to wear respirators. Alternatively, qualitative fit testing kits (Bitrix™) can be purchased for around $200.00.

When paired with a trained and competent fit test administrator (see 29 CFR 1910.134), these kits would allow cost-effective, on-site fit testing annually.

Conclusions

Trinity Rescue Mission needs to take steps to improve staff and volunteer training on symptoms of TB disease and prevention of disease transmission. Improved administrative procedures and policies need to be established and adopted at the shelter, to help identify guests displaying symptoms of TB disease or those listed on the DCHD target screening lists. Improved administrative controls would help reduce the potential for future cases of TB disease and help bring the ongoing outbreak under control. We also recommend that Trinity work more closely with DCHD representatives and use their expertise to help establish a comprehensive, written ICP for the shelter.

From an environmental control perspective, three of the four roof-top AHUs on the men's facility at the shelter were operational and capable of maintaining temperature and air flow, although there were issues with improper and inefficient filters. We were unable to verify the operability of AHU Men-4 serving the men's kitchen, since the unit was turned off during our visit. It was reported that the AHU is rarely used. All seven of the AHUs in the Women and Children's Center were adequately maintained and fully operational at the time of the NIOSH visit, but they also had low efficiency filters installed in each.

None of the AHUs at Trinity were providing fresh outdoor air to the occupied spaces, as required by the 2010 *Florida Building Code* and ASHRAE guidelines. Given the number of guests served by the shelter and the close proximity of guests to one another in most of the occupied spaces, it is important that these spaces are receiving adequate amounts of outdoor air. In addition to alleviating odors and better maintaining occupant comfort, outdoor air serves to dilute infectious aerosols, such as *M. tuberculosis* droplet nuclei responsible for TB transmission. With renovations, the existing AHUs might be made to provide the necessary outdoor air, or they could be augmented with the installation of new, dedicated outdoor air systems to provide the necessary outdoor air. A knowledgeable HVAC engineer should be consulted to discuss options for introducing outdoor air to the shelter.

The men's sleeping area houses 104 guests nearly every night. Given the occupant density, along with the benefit of the 15-feet ceiling height, a complete upper-room UVGI system should be installed in the space to further reduce the potential for airborne disease transmission. A qualified UVGI system designer or fixture manufacturer should be consulted for options. The system should be designed, operated, and maintained in accordance with applicable NIOSH guidelines. Once all changes and improvements to environmental controls at the shelter have been implemented, the shelter should develop a written preventive maintenance or O&M plan for the shelter.

For instances where improvements to administrative and environmental controls do not sufficiently mitigate the risk for disease transmission, respiratory protection might be necessary. There was no formal respiratory protection program in place during our visit, but such a program should be implemented at the shelter. Having this program in place will provide additional protection to Trinity staff and volunteers working in close proximity to guests with suspected TB or other airborne diseases. Any respirator use at the shelter should be covered by an OSHA-mandated respiratory protection program.

Essential improvements to administrative controls need to be made at Trinity to reduce the likelihood of future TB transmission at the shelter. Additionally, the environmental control systems need some attention to further reduce the risk. While ventilation systems and other environmental control systems cannot guarantee prevention of future TB disease transmission, improving the environmental controls will reduce the potential for airborne disease transmission, along with providing better indoor air quality throughout the shelter. The following recommendations are aimed at improving the overall infection control program at Trinity, with emphasis on improvements to environmental controls so they meet all applicable standards and guidelines.

Recommendations

Based on our assessment of environmental controls at Trinity Rescue Mission, we have developed the following list of recommendations, in order of priority:

1. **Improve and enhance the TB administrative controls at the shelter and develop a written Infection Control Plan.**

   - Work more closely with the DCHD to screen shelter staff, volunteers, and guests for TB disease.

   - With input from DCHD, develop specific procedures for handling a suspected or confirmed case of TB disease.

   - Educate shelter staff and volunteers on the signs and symptoms of TB disease so they can readily identify suspect cases and implement established precautions.

   - Consider displaying informational posters about TB signs and symptoms to educate guests.

   - Consider displaying signs encouraging proper cough etiquette and hand hygiene.

   - Develop a formal written TB Infection Control Plan. Seek guidance and input from DCHD and the Florida Department of Health. The plan should include:

     ○ All aspects of the TB infection control program and associated responsibilities, especially those functions requiring coordination with other agencies, such as the local and state health departments

     ○ All new and improved administrative controls put in place at Trinity

o Input from ventilation staff and/or guests tasked with servicing ventilation systems. Obtaining input from ventilation maintenance staff serves to strengthen the environmental control section of the plan while giving maintenance staff additional insight into the ventilation requirements for reducing or preventing airborne disease transmission.

o Schedule for updating and revising the ICP

2. **Introduce the required amounts of fresh outdoor air to all occupied spaces.**

- There are multiple options that can allow adequate outdoor air to be supplied to the shelter. All options, including the associated capital, maintenance, and annual operating costs should be considered. Work with a reputable ventilation or engineering contractor familiar with the current *Florida Building Code*, ASHRAE, FGI, and CDC guidelines to select the best option for Trinity.

- Improve air flow patterns within all occupied spaces, particularly the men's sleeping area and the women's overnight room. Air flow patterns should provide effective ventilation and temperature control while minimizing the number of people that air travels across before returning to the AHU.

3. **Improve filtration efficiency in all AHUs.** Select higher efficiency filters (higher MERV ratings) for use in each AHU, as long as the new filters do not adversely impact the required air flow delivery capacity of the AHUs.

4. **Create a respiratory separation area in the men's sleeping area.**

- Choose a reputable ventilation or engineering design contractor that is familiar with current *Florida Building Code*, ASHRAE, FGI, and CDC guidelines and recommendations. Ideally a small room should be constructed in a corner of the sleeping area specifically for respiratory separation. If construction of a separate room is impractical, a less-desirable approach is to install impervious retractable partitions that could be used to enclose a corner of the men's sleeping area when respiratory separation is warranted. The partitions should touch the floor and extend as close to the ceiling as possible. While there are various ways to develop a respiratory separation area, it should include the following:

  o Ensure that all supply and return ductwork for the AHU serving the newly-constructed room or area enclosed by partitions is intact and sealed. Install tight-sealing return dampers on each return from the selected transition room to eliminate return air flow when the space is used for respiratory separation. Ensure that supply air diffusers provide good air mixing and air flow patterns in a newly-constructed room.

- o Design and install an auxiliary exhaust system that enables the respiratory separation area to be maintained under negative pressure when housing guests for separation purposes. One approach to this requirement would be to select and install exhaust fans directly through the outside walls of the rooms. The fans can be mounted through the walls themselves or mounted on the roof with ductwork through the walls to the fans.

- o Install the highest efficiency air filters in the AHU that will still allow adequate airflow to meet the AHU's conditioning requirements. Adjust and balance the system as necessary to ensure proper air flows at all times when the room or curtain enclosure is used for respiratory separation and normal purposes. Ensure that adequate outdoor air is supplied to each space at all times (see Recommendation 2 above).

- o Develop a detailed written plan for the conversion of the room or partition enclosure from normal housing functions to use for respiratory separation. The plan should include:

  - Procedures for moving the guests currently in these areas to other locations
  - Procedures for cleaning and refurnishing the areas for separation purposes, and step-by-step procedures for staff to follow to start the exhaust fan, close the return air dampers, and test for negative pressure
  - Measures for preparing the areas for back-to-back occupants requiring separation
  - Procedures for cleaning and returning the areas to normal use after the need for respiratory separation has passed

- o Operate the new systems as designed and according to the written plan. When in use, the respiratory separation area should be visually tested with smoke tubes or flutter strips daily to ensure negative pressure is being maintained while the room is occupied for separation. When the area is being used for normal purposes, it should be tested monthly to ensure proper operation in the event it would be needed for respiratory separation. The results of all pressure testing should be documented.

5. **Modify at least one bedroom on the first floor of the women's shelter into a respiratory separation area.**

- Choose a reputable ventilation or engineering design contractor that is familiar with current *Florida Building Code*, ASHRAE, FGI, and CDC guidelines and recommendations. While there are various ways to develop a respiratory separation area, it should include the following:

- o Ensure that all supply and return ductwork for the AHU serving the selected room is intact and sealed. Install tight-sealing return dampers on each return from the selected room to eliminate return air flow when the space is used for respiratory separation. Ensure that supply air diffusers provide good air mixing and air flow patterns in each selected room.

- o Design and install an auxiliary exhaust system that enables the respiratory separation area to be maintained under negative pressure when housing guests for separation purposes. One approach to this requirement would be to select and install exhaust fans directly through the outside walls of the rooms. The fans can be mounted through the walls themselves or mounted on the roof with ductwork through the walls to the fans. Fan design/placement should ensure that the adjacent bathroom stays under negative pressure when the bedroom is used for respiratory separation purposes.

- o Install the highest efficiency air filters in the AHU that will still allow adequate airflow to meet the AHU's conditioning requirements. Adjust and balance the system as necessary to ensure proper air flows at all times when each selected room is individually or collectively used for respiratory separation and normal purposes. Ensure that adequate outdoor air is supplied to each space at all times (see Recommendation 2 above).

- o Develop a detailed written plan for the conversion of the selected room(s) from normal housing functions to use for respiratory separation. The plan should include:

  - Procedures for moving the guests currently in these areas to other locations
  - Procedures for cleaning and refurnishing the areas for separation purposes, and step-by-step procedures for staff to follow to start the exhaust fan, close the return air dampers, and test for negative pressure
  - Measures for preparing the areas for back-to-back occupants requiring separation
  - Procedures for cleaning and returning the areas to normal use after the need for respiratory separation has passed

- o Operate the new systems as designed and according to the written plan. When in use, the respiratory separation area should be visually tested with smoke tubes or flutter strips daily to ensure negative pressure is being maintained while the room is occupied for separation. When the room is being used for normal purposes, it should be tested monthly to ensure proper operation in the event it would be needed for respiratory separation. The results of all pressure testing should be documented.

6. **Install an upper-room UVGI system in the men's sleeping area.**

   - Choose a qualified UVGI fixture manufacturer or system engineer, familiar with the NIOSH upper-room guidelines, to design, install and test the system. The system designer/installer should also provide initial training on exposure hazards, safety, and system maintenance.

   - The system should be designed to provide UV irradiance levels of at least 30–50 $\mu W/cm^2$ in the upper portion of the room while limiting UVC exposure to occupants in the area to a level below the NIOSH REL for UVC of 6.0 mJ/cm^2 for an 8-hour exposure time.

   - Operate the upper-room UVGI system all day, every day, or at least at all times the men's sleeping area is occupied.

   - Establish a UVGI safety, operation, and maintenance program.

   - Conduct training and maintenance in accordance with NIOSH guidelines and/or applicable manufacturer recommendations.

7. **Make necessary ventilation changes so clinic examination rooms in the women's shelter are properly maintained under negative pressure in relation to the adjacent waiting area.** Negative pressure might be established by adjusting existing dampers or ductwork so more air is exhausted from the exam rooms than is being supplied to them. If negative pressure cannot be maintained with such adjustments, the installation of separate exhaust fans from each space may be required. If new exhaust fans are required, they should be operated any time the examination rooms are occupied.

8. **Develop and implement an OSHA respiratory protection program in accordance with 29 CFR 1910.134.** To meet the OSHA requirements, you must:

   - Designate a program administrator who is qualified by appropriate training or experience to administer or oversee the program and conduct the required program evaluations.

   - Provide respirators, training, and medical evaluations at no cost to employees or staff required to wear respirators on the job.

   - Develop a written program with worksite-specific procedures when respirators are necessary or required by the employer. The written respiratory protection program needs to include:

- Respirator types and proper respirator selection
- Required medical evaluations for employees prior to respirator use
- Procedures for initial and annual respirator fit testing
- Instructions for proper respirator use
- Information on appropriate respirator maintenance and care
- Initial and yearly training requirements for respirator users
- Procedures for evaluating the effectiveness of the respiratory protection program
- Update the respiratory protection program as necessary to reflect changes in workplace conditions that affect respirator use.

9. **Repair all non-functional bathroom exhaust fans or install new ones.** Ensure that air is being exhausted from each bathroom and shower facility and that each area is under negative pressure, in accordance with the 2010 *Florida Building Code* and ASHRAE requirements. Ensure that all exhaust air from bathrooms and shower facilities is exhausted directly outside and that no return air from bathrooms is recirculated back to an AHU or entrained in the outdoor air entering any current or future AHU.

10. **After all of the ventilation systems are updated and functioning properly, develop a comprehensive, written HVAC O&M plan.** The O&M Plan should include:

- Preventive maintenance schedules and all regularly scheduled maintenance tasks (filter changes, fan belt inspections, UV lamp changes, etc.) and who is responsible for conducting each task
- Written procedures for each maintenance task to ensure the work is done properly each time, regardless of who performs the work.
- Training requirements for maintenance staff
- A method for logging maintenance activities for each AHU
- A method for updating or revising the O&M Plan as procedures or systems change

Outline of Future NIOSH Involvement

This report will serve to close out NIOSH Technical Assistance at Trinity. However, we understand that the work outlined in the recommendations above will take several months to complete and will represent a significant investment of time and financial resources. As the work proceeds, NIOSH could assist by:

- Reviewing any Requests for Proposal developed to initiate the bidding process
- Reviewing any bids received in response to Requests for Proposals for technical content
- Providing technical assistance related to any environmental control strategies, including upper-room UVGI systems

It is not necessary for NIOSH to be on-site during any ventilation renovations. Yet, as projects are initiated, we can assist you by reviewing:

- Proposed modification strategies for outdoor air introduction or respiratory separation area designs
- Preliminary design schematics or equipment selection documents
- Air flow testing and balancing reports
- Final project documents, including as-built drawings, sequences of operations, and proper equipment set points

Once the renovations are complete, if additional NIOSH assistance is desired or warranted, the request for technical assistance can be reopened.

References

ACGIH (American Conference of Governmental Industrial Hygienists) [2012]. Threshold limit values for chemical substances and physical agents & biological exposure indicies. Cincinnati, OH: American Conference of Governmental Industrial Hygienists.

ANSI/ASHRAE (American National Standards Institute/American Society of Heating, Ventilating and Air-Conditioning Engineers) [2007]. Method of testing general ventilation air-cleaning devices for removal efficiency by particle size. Atlanta, GA: American Society of Heating, Refrigerating and Air-Conditioning Engineers. Standard 52.2-2007.

ANSI/ASHRAE [2010a]. Ventilation for acceptable indoor air quality. Atlanta, GA: American Society of Heating, Refrigerating and Air-Conditioning Engineers. Standard 62.1-2010.

ANSI/ASHRAE [2010b]. Thermal environmental conditions for human occupancy. Atlanta, GA: American Society of Heating, Refrigerating and Air-Conditioning Engineers. Standard 55-2010.

ASHRAE [2011]. Ultraviolet air and surface treatment. In: ASHRAE Handbook – HVAC Applications, Chapter 60. Atlanta, GA: American Society of Heating, Refrigerating and Air-Conditioning Engineers.

ASHRAE [2012]. Ultraviolet lamp systems. In: ASHRAE Handbook – HVAC Systems and Equipment, Chapter 17. Atlanta, GA: American Society of Heating, Refrigerating and Air-Conditioning Engineers.

Barry MA, Wall C, Shirley L, Bernardo J, Schwingl P, Brigandi E, Lamb GA [1986]. Tuberculosis screening in Boston's homeless shelters. Public Health Rep *101*(5):487-498.

Brickner PW, Vincent RL, First M, Nardell E, Murray M, Kaufman W [2003]. The application of ultraviolet germicidal irradiation to control transmission of airborne disease: bioterrorism countermeasure. Public Health Rep 118:99-118.

CDC (Centers for Disease Control and Prevention) [1985]. Drug-resistant tuberculosis among the homeless—Boston. MMWR *34*:429-431.

CDC [1992]. Prevention and control of tuberculosis among homeless persons (ACET). MMWR *41*(RR-5):001.

CDC [2003a]. Tuberculosis outbreak in a homeless population—Portland, Maine, 2002-2003. MMWR *52*(48):1184-1185.

CDC [2003b]. TB outbreak among homeless persons—King County, Washington, 2002-2003. MMWR *52*(49):1209-1210.

CDC [2005a]. Tuberculosis transmission in a homeless shelter population—New York, 2000-2003. MMWR 54(06):149-152.

CDC [2005b]. Guidelines for preventing the transmission of *Mycobacterium tuberculosis* in health-care settings, 2005. MMWR 54(RR-17):1-141.

CDC [2006]. Prevention and control of tuberculosis in correctional and detention facilities: Recommendations from CDC. MMWR 55(RR-9):1-54.

David HL [1973]. Response of mycobacteria to ultraviolet light radiation. Am Rev Respir Dis 108:1175-85.

EPA (US Environmental Protection Agency) [2012]. The inside story: A guide to indoor air quality http://www.epa.gov/iaq/pubs/insidestory.html. Date accessed: February 22, 2013.

FGI (Facility Guidelines Institute) [2010]. Guidelines for design and construction of health care facilities. Chicago, IL: American Society for Healthcare Engineering of the American Hospital Association.

First MW, Nardell EA, Chaisson W, Riley R [1999a]. Guidelines for the application of upper-room ultraviolet germicidal irradiation for preventing transmission of airborne contagion - part I: basic principles. ASHRAE Trans 105(1):CH-99-12-91.

First MW, Nardell EA, Chaisson W, Riley R [1999b]. Guidelines for the application of upper-room ultraviolet germicidal irradiation for preventing transmission of airborne contagion - Part II: design and operation guidance. ASHRAE Trans 105(1):CH-99-12-92.

ICC (International Code Council, Inc.) [2011]. Florida building code 2010: Mechanical (chapter 4, ventilation). Country Club Hills, IL: International Code Council, Inc.

Knopf SA [1914]. Tuberculosis as a cause and result of poverty. J Am Med Assoc 63(20):1720-1725.

McAdam JM, Brickner PW, Scharer LL, Crocco JA, Duff AE [1990]. The spectrum of tuberculosis in a New York City men's shelter clinic (1982-1988). Chest 97:798-805.

McLean RL [1961]. General discussion: the mechanism of spread of Asian influenza. Am Rev Respir Dis 83:29-40.

NIOSH [1972]. Criteria for a recommended standard: occupational exposures to ultraviolet radiation. By Seiter RE. Cincinnati, OH: U.S. Department of Health, Education, and Welfare, Health Services and Mental Health Administration, National Institute for Occupational Safety and Health, DHEW (NIOSH) Publication No. HSM-73-11009.

NIOSH [2009]. Environmental control for tuberculosis: basic upper-room ultraviolet germicidal irradiation guidelines for healthcare settings. By Whalen J. Cincinnati, OH: U.S. Department of Health and Human Services, Centers for Disease Control and Prevention, National Institute for Occupational Safety and Health, DHHS (NIOSH)

Publication No. 2009-105. http://www.cdc.gov/niosh/docs/2009-105/pdfs/2009-105.pdf. Date accessed: March 22, 2013.

Nolan CM, Elarth AM, Barr H, Saeed AM, Risser DR [1991]. An outbreak of tuberculosis in a shelter for homeless men: A description of its evolution and control. Am Rev Respir Dis *143*:257-261.

Riley RL, Wells WF, Mills CC, Nyka W, McLean RL [1957]. Air hygiene in tuberculosis: quantitative studies of infectivity and control in a pilot ward. Am Rev Tubercul 75:420-31.

Riley RL, Mills CC, O'Grady F, Sultan LU, Wittstadt F, Shivpuri DN [1962]. Infectiousness of air from a tuberculosis ward. Am Rev Respir Dis 85:511-25.

Riley RL, Knight M, Middlebrook G [1976]. Ultraviolet susceptibility of BCG and virulent tubercle bacilli. Am Rev Respir Dis 113:413-18.

Riley RL, Nardell EA [1989]. Clearing the air: the theory and application of ultraviolet air disinfection. Am Rev Respir Dis 139(5):1286-94.

Slutkin G [1986]. Management of tuberculosis in urban homeless indigents. Public Health Rep *101*(5):481-485.

Wells WF, Holla, WA [1950]. Ventilation in the flow of measles and chickenpox through a community: progress report, January 1, 1946 to June 15, 1949—airborne infection study, Westchester County department of health. J Am Med Assoc 142:1337-44.

Willmon TL, Hollaender A, Langmuir AD [1948]. Studies of the control of acute respiratory diseases among naval recruits. I. a review of a four-year experience with ultraviolet irradiation and dust suppressive measures, 1943 to 1947. Am J Hyg 48:227-32.

Xu P, Peccia J, Fabian P, Martyny JW, Fennelly KP, Hernandez M, Miller SL [2003]. Efficacy of ultraviolet germicidal irradiation of upper-room air in inactivating airborne bacterial spores and mycobacteria in full-scale studies. Atmos Environ 37:405-19.

Tables

Table 1. General air-handling unit (AHU) information

NIOSH AHU Identifier	Physical Location of AHU	Location Served by AHU (floor/building)[A]	AHU Manufacturer[B]	AHU Model Number[B]	Proper Filter Configuration in AHU[C,D]	Actual Filter Configuration in AHU[B,D,E]
Men-1	Rooftop of Men's Facility	Men's Sleeping Area	Carrier	50HJQ012	(4) $20 \times 20 \times 2$	*(4) $18 \times 14 \times 2$[F]
Men-2	Rooftop of Men's Facility	Men's Facility Chapel Area	Carrier	50TJQ008	(4) $16 \times 20 \times 2$	*(4) $18 \times 14 \times 2$[F]
Men-3	Rooftop of Men's Facility	Men's Facility Dining Area	Goodman	CPH090XXX3BXXXAA	(4) $16 \times 24 \times 2$	(4) $16 \times 24 \times 2$
Men-4	Rooftop of Men's Facility	Men's Facility Kitchen	Carrier	50TJQ012	(4) $20 \times 20 \times 2$	*(4) $18 \times 14 \times 2$[F]
Women-1[G]	Women's Facility (1st Floor Mechanical Room)	Women's Facility (1st Floor/ Undetermined)[H]	Carrier	40RMQ016	(4) $16 \times 24 \times 2$ and (4) $16 \times 20 \times 2$	(4) $16 \times 24 \times 2$ and (4) $16 \times 20 \times 2$
Women-2[G]	Women's Facility (1st Floor Mechanical Room)	Women's Facility (1st Floor/ Undetermined)[H]	Carrier	FK4DNF003	(1) $21 \times 20 \times 1$	(1) $21 \times 20 \times 1$
Women-3[G]	Women's Facility (1st Floor Mechanical Room)	Women's Facility (1st Floor/ Undetermined)[H]	Carrier	FK4DNF005	(1) $21 \times 20 \times 1$	(1) $21 \times 20 \times 1$
Women-4[G]	Women's Facility (Attic)	Women's Facility (2nd Floor/ Rooms 18-19, D2, and laundry room)[I]	Carrier	FK4DNB006	(1) $21 \times 24 \times 1$	(1) $21 \times 24 \times 1$
Women-5[G]	Women's Facility (Attic)	Women's Facility (2nd Floor/ Rooms 14-17 and partially showers/ restroom)[I]	Carrier	FK4DNF003	(1) $21 \times 20 \times 1$	(1) $21 \times 20 \times 1$
Women-6[G]	Women's Facility (Attic)	Women's Facility (2nd Floor/ Rooms 10-13 and partially showers/ restroom)[I]	Carrier	FK4DNF005	(1) $21 \times 20 \times 1$	(1) $21 \times 20 \times 1$
Women-7[G]	Women's Facility (Attic)	Women's Facility (2nd Floor/ Rooms 7-9 and D1)[I]	Carrier	FK4DNB006	(1) $21 \times 24 \times 1$	(1) $21 \times 24 \times 1$

[A] May not represent all locations served by the AHU

[B] Information taken during visual inspection of AHU

[C] Information gathered from product data specific to each AHU model published by respective AHU manufacturer.

[D] Value in parenthesis represents the number of filters; dimensions are width × height × depth in units of inches

[E] Entries preceded by an asterisk (*) represent actual filter configurations that differ from published proper filter configurations. Differences could be due to incorrect filter size(s) being installed or because the AHU manufacturer modified the AHU model size/filter recommendation as the product was updated.

[F] Filters in this AHU appeared to be homemade and not commercially available. Therefore, no information on filter performance was available.

[G] All supply ductwork from the AHU was wrapped in fiberglass.

[H] It was not determined which AHU(s) supplied air to individual spaces on the first floor of the Women's Facility. Doing so would have required unfettered access to thermo stats and/or removing multiple ceiling tiles. This would have caused a significant disruption to staff and guests on the first floor at the time.

[I] The locations served by the 2nd floor AHUs in the Women's Facility was determined by turning various thermostats on and off. Information may not be entirely correct.

Table 2. Applicable outdoor air supply flow rates, minimum exhaust air flow rates, and default occupancy densities from the *2010 Florida Building Code and ASHRAE Standard 62.1-2010*[A]

Occupancy Category	People Outdoor Air Flow Rate (cfm/person)[B]	Area Outdoor Air Flow Rate (cfm/ft^2)[C]	Minimum Exhaust Air Flow Rate[D]	Default Occupant Density (#/1000 ft^2)[E]
Barracks/Dormitory Sleeping Areas	5	0.06	—	20
Bedrooms/Living Rooms	5	0.06	—	10
Office Spaces	5	0.06	—	5
Conference Rooms	5	0.06	—	50
Multipurpose Assembly Spaces	5	0.06	—	120
Reception Areas	5	0.06	—	30
Break Rooms[F]	5[F]	0.12[F]	—	50[F]
Central Laundry Rooms[F]	5[F]	0.12[F]	—	10[F]
Occupiable Dry Storage Rooms[F]	5[F]	0.06[F]	—	2[F]
Occupiable Liquid/Gel Storage Rooms[F]	5[F]	0.12[F]	—	2[F]
Unoccupiable Storage Rooms[G]	—	0.12[G]	—	—
Lobbies/Prefunction Spaces	7.5	0.06	—	30
Lecture Classrooms	7.5	0.06	—	65
Computer Labs	10	0.12	—	25
Dining Rooms	7.5	0.18	—	70
Central Kitchens	7.5[F]	0.12[F]	0.7 cfm/ft^2[C]	70
Public Bathrooms	—	—	50 or 70 cfm/toilet and/or urinal[H]	—
Private Bathrooms	—	—	25 or 50 cfm[I]	—
Shower Rooms[G]	—	—	20 or 50 cfm/shower head[G,J]	—

[A] Requirements published in: *2010 Florida Building Code: Mechanical* (Chapter 4, Ventilation). International Code Council, Inc., Country Club Hills, IL (2011) and American National Standards Institute (ANSI)/American Society of Heating, Refrigerating and Air-Conditioning Engineers (ASHRAE). *Ventilation for Acceptable Indoor Air Quality,* Standard 62.1-2010. ASHRAE, Atlanta, GA (2010). In nearly all cases, the *2010 Florida Building Code* has adopted ventilation recommendations directly from ASHRAE Standard 62.1-2010.

[B] cfm/person = cubic feet per minute (also commonly shown as ft^3/min) per person typically in the occupied space

[C] cfm/ft^2 = cubic feet per minute (also commonly shown as ft^3/min) per square feet of occupied space

[D] Mechanical exhaust should be released directly outdoors at least 25 feet away from air intakes. Recirculation of exhaust air back into the building should be avoided.

[E] #/1000ft^2 = number of people per 1000 square feet of occupied space. These values are typical occupant densities in spaces that are useful for building/HVAC system design. If actual occupant densities are known, they should be used instead of these default values.

[F] Requirements are only published in ASHRAE Standard 62.1-2010. No directly corresponding values appear in the *2010 Florida Building Code.*

[G] Requirements are only published in the *2010 Florida Building Code.* No directly corresponding values appear in ASHRAE Standard 62.1-2010.

[H] Provide the higher rate when periods of heavy use are expected to occur (e.g. prior to guests leaving in the morning). If periods of heavy use are not antici pated, the lower rate may be used.

[I] These rates are for bathrooms intended for use by one person at a time. If exhaust fans are operated continuously, the lower rate may be used. If exhaust fans are operated intermittently (e.g., fans activated by a light switch), the higher rate should be used.

[J] If exhaust fans are operated continuously, the lower rate may be used. If exhaust fans are operated intermittently (e.g., fans activated by a light switch), the higher rate should be used.

Table 3. Total air delivered by ventilation systems, occupant densities, and recommended outdoor air flow

Space[A]	AHU Serving Space	Return Flow from Space (cfm)[B]	Supply Flow into Space (cfm)[B]	Approximate Area of Space (ft²)[C]	Typical Occupants in Space[D]	Occupant Density (#/1000 ft²)[D,E,F]	Recommended Outdoor Air Flow (cfm)[B,G]
Men's Facility							
Reception/Lobby Area	Undetermined[H]	<30[I]	130	390	3	8	38.4
Sleeping Area	Men-1	2435	3110	2530	104	*41	671.8
Bathroom/Showers off Sleeping Area	Men-1	520	0[I]	440	N/A[J]	N/A[J]	N/A[J]
Chapel/Dining Area	Men-2 (chapel) and Men-3 (dining)	3680	4410	3105	140	45	886.3/1608.9[K]
1st Floor – Women's Facility							
Reception/Lobby Area and Hallway	Undetermined[H]	285	890	1220	2	2	83.2
Dining Area/Classroom	Undetermined[H]	300	1245	940	30	32	206.4/394.2[K]
Play Room	Undetermined[H]	130	150	425	4	9	45.5
Restroom in Play Room	Undetermined[H]	0[I]	40	65	N/A[J]	N/A[J]	N/A[J]
Clinic Waiting Area	Undetermined[H]	260	40	95	2	21	15.7
Clinic Office	Undetermined[H]	115	80	45	1	22	7.7
Clinic Exam Room #1[L]	Undetermined[H]	0[I]	70	80	2	25	14.8
Clinic Exam Room #2[L]	Undetermined[H]	Obs[M]	50	70	2	29	14.2
Clinic Back Room/Storage	Undetermined[H]	160	70	35	0	0	4.2
Clinic Restroom	Undetermined[H]	0[I]	70	40	N/A[J]	N/A[J]	N/A[J]
Women's Overnight Sleeping Room	Undetermined[H]	470	570	505	18	*36	120.3
Women's Overnight Restroom	Undetermined[H]	0[I]	0[I]	75	N/A[J]	N/A[J]	N/A[J]
Room #1	Undetermined[H]	50	105	195	1	5	16.7
Room #1 Bathroom	Undetermined[H]	0[I]	0[I]	30	N/A[N]	N/A[N]	N/A[N]
Room #2	Undetermined[H]	95	140	195	5	*26	36.7
Room #2 Bathroom	Undetermined[H]	0[I]	0[I]	30	N/A[N]	N/A[N]	N/A[N]
Room #3	Undetermined[H]	40	130	195	1	5	16.7
Room #3 Bathroom	Undetermined[H]	0[I]	0[I]	30	N/A[N]	N/A[N]	N/A[N]
Room #4	Undetermined[H]	110	180	195	4	*21	31.7
Room #4 Bathroom	Undetermined[H]	0[I]	0[I]	30	N/A[N]	N/A[N]	N/A[N]
Room #5	Undetermined[H]	100	140	230	3	13	28.8

Table 3 (continued). Total air delivered by ventilation systems, occupant densities, and recommended outdoor air flow

Space[A]	AHU Serving Space	Return Flow from Space (cfm)[B]	Supply Flow into Space (cfm)[B]	Approximate Area of Space (ft²)[C]	Typical Occupants in Space[D]	Occupant Density (#/1000 ft²)[D,E,F]	Recommended Outdoor Air Flow (cfm)[B,G]
1st Floor – Women's Facility							
Room #5 Bathroom	Undetermined[H]	0[I]	0[I]	35	N/A[N]	N/A[N]	N/A[N]
Room #6	Undetermined[H]	110	170	195	2	10	21.7
Room #6 Bathroom	Undetermined[H]	0[I]	0[I]	65	N/A[N]	N/A[N]	N/A[N]
2nd Floor – Women's Facility							
Room D1	Women-7[O]	440	540	805	12	15	108.3
Room #7	Women-7[O]	155	160	240	4	17	34.4
Room #8	Women-7[O]	155	175	240	4	17	34.4
Room #9	Women-7[O]	140	225	240	4	17	34.4
Room #10	Women-6[O]	130	130	240	4	17	34.4
Room #11	Women-6[O]	130	190	240	4	17	34.4
Room #12	Women-6[O]	160	195	240	4	17	34.4
Room #13	Women-6[O]	135	180	240	4	17	34.4
Room #14	Women-5[O]	135	210	240	4	17	34.4
Room #15	Women-5[O]	140	215	240	4	17	34.4
Room #16	Women-5[O]	125	170	240	4	17	34.4
Room #17	Women-5[O]	140	230	240	4	17	34.4
Room #18	Women-4[O]	120	200	240	4	17	34.4
Room #19	Women-4[O]	240	200	240	4	17	34.4
Room D2	Women-4[O]	580	260	370	6	16	52.2
Showers and Restroom	Women-5 & Women-6[O]	720	575	945	N/A[J]	N/A[J]	N/A[J]
Laundry Room	Women-4[O]	795	335	240	1	4	33.8

[A] May not represent all locations served by the AHU
[B] cfm = cubic feet per minute (also commonly shown as ft³/min)
[C] ft² = square feet
[D] Occupant numbers estimated by visual observation during NIOSH visit
[E] #/1000 ft² = number of occupants per 1000 ft² of occupied floor space. Calculated by dividing the number of typical occupants in the space by the approximate area of the space and multiplying by 1000

F Entries preceded by an asterisk (*) represent spaces where the actual occupant density likely exceeds the default occupant density presented in Table 2.

G Calculated based on recommendations published in: American National Standards Institute (ANSI)/American Society of Heating, Refrigerating and Air-Conditioning Engineers (ASHRAE). Ventilation for Acceptable Indoor Air Quality, Standard 62.1-2010. ASHRAE, Atlanta, GA (2010). ASHRAE, Atlanta, GA (2010) and the *2010 Florida Building Code: Mechanical* (Chapter 4, Ventilation). International Code Council, Inc., Country Club Hills, IL (2011). In nearly all cases, the *2010 Florida Building Code* has adopted ventilation recommendations directly from ASHRAE Standard 62.1-2010.

H It was not determined which AHU(s) supplied air to this space. Doing so would have required unfettered access to thermostats and/or removing multiple ceiling tiles. This would have caused a significant disruption to staff and guests on the first floor at the time.

I A TSI Accubalance Plus, Model 8373, was used to determine air flow measurements. The instrument is unable to accurately read volumetric air flow rates less than 30 cfm. Reading could be anywhere between 0 and 30 cfm. In these cases, ventilation fog was used to visually determine if any air was flowing through the vent/grille. When there was visual confirmation of air flow, the result was reported as < 30 cfm. When air flow could not be verified visually, the result was reported as 0 cfm.

J N/A = not applicable. Neither ASHRAE Standard 62.1-2010 nor the *2010 Florida Building Code* include outdoor air recommendations for restrooms, bathrooms, and shower facili ties. Instead, for public bathrooms, the recommendation is 50 cfm of exhaust from the space per toilet or urinal when periods of heavy use are not expected. ASHRAE 62.1-2010 does not specifically address ventilation for showers. However, the *2010 Florida Building Code: Mechanical* (Chapter 4, Ventilation) specifies 50 cfm of exhaust air from the space per shower head when the exhaust system is designed to operate intermittently (e.g., exhaust fan connected to light switch) or 20 cfm per shower head for exhaust systems designed to operate continuously. Water closet and shower exhaust may be made up entirely of transfer air from adjacent spaces (i.e., no direct supply air to the space is required) and only a maximum of 10% of the exhaust air is permitted to be recycled.

K ASHRAE Standard 62.1-2010 and the *2010 Florida Building Code: Mechanical* (Chapter 4, Ventilation) provide separate outdoor air recommendations for assembly spaces and dining rooms. Both numbers are reported here (assembly space/dining area).

L Areas where medical examinations and/or procedures are performed should be maintained under negative pressure compared to adjacent areas (i.e., more air should be exhausted from the space than is supplied to the space). Exam Room #1 was under positive pressure during the NIOSH visit. The pressure relationship between inside and outside of Exam Room #2 was not determined.

M Obs = obstructed. Air flow measurements could not be taken because the exhaust grille was obstructed. Exhaust was determined to be working via ventilation fog testing.

N N/A = not applicable. Living areas on the first floor of the Women's Facility are equipped with private bathrooms. ASHRAE Standard 62.1-2010 and the *2010 Florida Building Code: Mechanical* (Chapter 4, Ventilation) specifies 25 cfm of exhaust air per toilet. This exhaust air may be made up entirely of transfer air from adjacent spaces (i.e., no direct supply air to the space is required) and only a maximum of 10% of the exhaust air is permitted to be recycled.

O The locations served by the 2nd floor AHUs in the Women's Facility were determined by turning various thermostats on and off. Information may not be entirely correct.

Table 4. ASHRAE indoor relative humidity and temperature recommendations[A]

Relative Humidity	Winter Temperatures[B]	Summer Temperatures[B]
30%[C]	69.5°F to 77.0°F	75.5°F to 81.5°F
40%	69.0°F to 76.5°F	75.5°F to 81.0°F
50%[D]	68.5°F to 76.0°F	75.0°F to 80.5°F

[A] Adapted from: American National Standards Institute (ANSI)/American Society of Heating, Refrigerating and Air-Conditioning Engineers (ASHRAE). Thermal Environmental Conditions for Human Occupancy, Standard 55-2010. ASHRAE, Atlanta, GA. (2010).
[B] Applies to occupants wearing typical summer and winter clothing, with a sedentary to light activity level
[C] Humidity levels below 30% may cause irritated mucus membranes, dry eyes, and sinus discomfort.
[D] The U.S. Environmental Protection Agency recommends maintaining indoor relative humidity below 60% and ideally in a range from 30% to 50% to prevent mold growth.

Figures

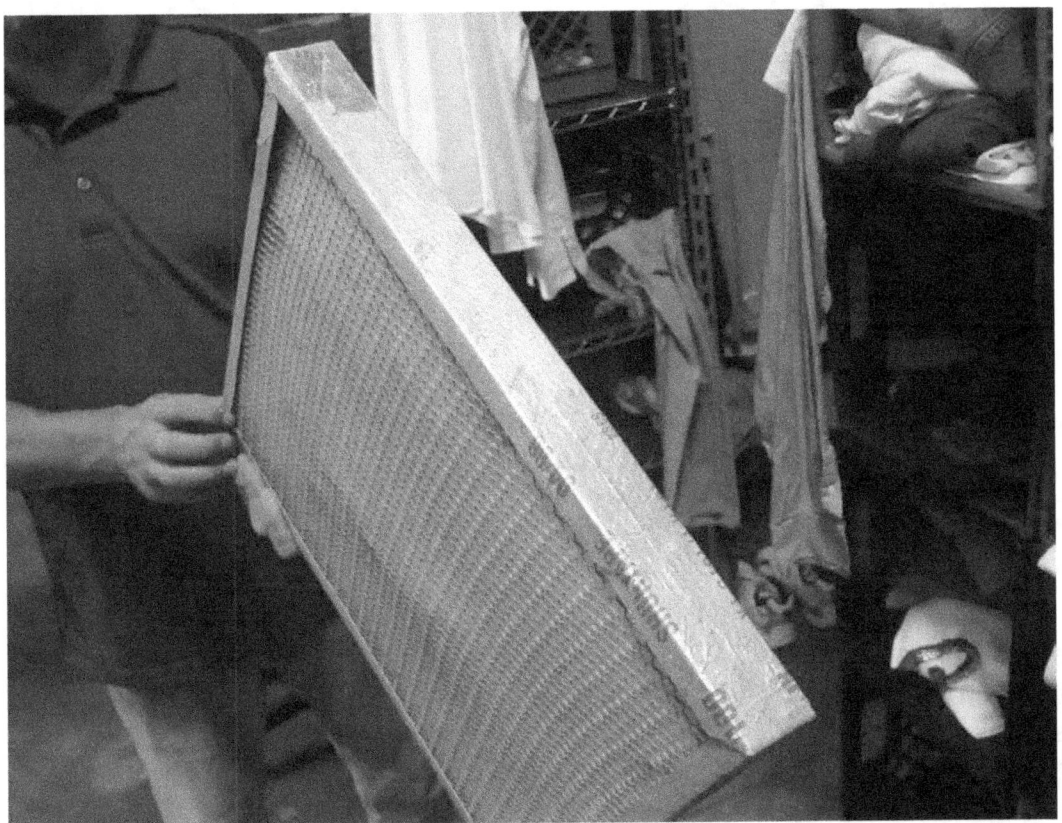

Figure 1. A represnentative ventilation filter from inside AHU Men-1, AHU Men -2, and AHU Men-4.

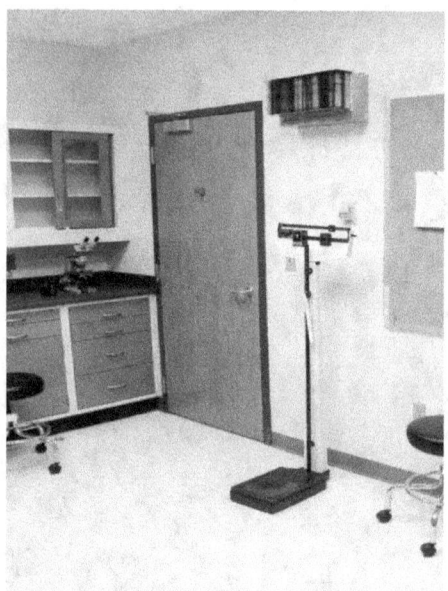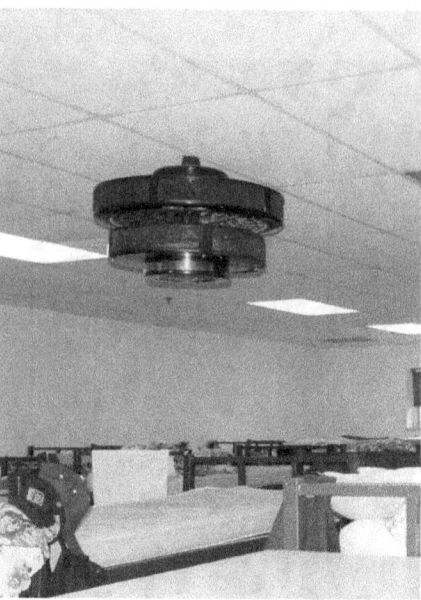

Figure 2. Typical upper-air UVGI installations: Left–Wall-mounted fixture with louvers installed in a health clinic; Right–Ceiling-mounted fixture with a fan installed in a homeless shelter.

The Health Hazard Evaluation Program investigates possible health hazards in the workplace under the authority of Section 20(a)(6) of the Occupational Safety and Health Act of 1970, 29 U.S.C. 669(a)(6). The Health Hazard Evaluation Program also provides, upon request, technical assistance to federal, state, and local agencies to control occupational health hazards and to prevent occupational illness and disease. Regulations guiding the Program can be found in Title 42, Code of Federal Regulations, Part 85; Requests for Health Hazard Evaluations (42 CFR 85).

Acknowledgments

This report was prepared by Stephen B. Martin, Jr., R. Brent Lawrence, and Michael C. Beaty of the Field Studies Branch (FSB), Division of Respiratory Disease Studies (DRDS) and Kenneth R. Mead of the Engineering and Physical Hazards Branch, Division of Applied Research and Technology. Desktop publishing was performed by Tia McClelland (FSB/DRDS).

Availability of Report

Copies of this report have been sent to representatives from Trinity Rescue Mission, DCHD, the Florida Department of Health, CDC/NCHHSTP/DTBE, and the OSHA Regional Office. This report is not copyrighted and may be freely reproduced.

This report is available at http://www.cdc.gov/niosh/hhe/reports/pdfs/2012-0265-3183.pdf.

Recommended citation for this report:
NIOSH [2013]. Health hazard evaluation report: EEvaluation of Environmental Controls at a Homeless Shelter (Trinity Rescue Mission) Associated with a Tuberculosis Outbreak – Florida. By Martin, Jr. SB, Mead KR, Lawrence RB, Beaty MC. Morgantown, WV: U.S. Department of Health and Human Services, Centers for Disease Control and Prevention, National Institute for Occupational Safety and Health, NIOSH Report No. 2012-0265-3183.